Father,

Thank you for the abilities you give us, for the strength and wisdom we gain from training.

Be with us as we work that we may do our best. Help us to be encouraging to others in our daily life. Thank you for the people that you have brought into our lives.

Bless the athletes, coaches, workout partners and all those who support our training.
May the results from our training be a reflection of Your Spirit in our lives.

Finally Father, remind us that there is no failure, but only growth in the body, mind and Spirit.

Amen

Contents

Copyright

Bodyweight Cross Training WOD Bible: 220 Travel Friendly Home Workouts

First Edition – April 2014.

Written by P Selter

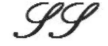

A Shredded-Society Publication
www.Shredded-Society.com
Copyright © 2014
All rights reserved.

Disclaimer

The information provided in this book is designed to provide helpful information on the subjects discussed. This book is not meant to be used, nor should it be used, to diagnose or treat any medical condition. For diagnosis or treatment of any medical problem, consult your own physician. The publisher and author are not responsible for any specific health or allergy needs that may require medical supervision and are not liable for any damages or negative consequences from any treatment, action, application or preparation, to any person reading or following the information in this book. References are provided for informational purposes only and do not constitute endorsement of any websites or other sources. Readers should be aware that the websites listed in this book may change.

I recommend consulting a doctor to assess and/or identify any health related issues prior to making any dramatic changes to your diet or exercise regime.

Bonus Content

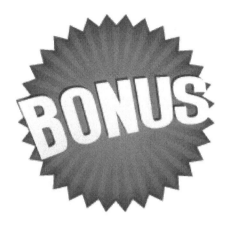

As a token of our appreciation Shredded-Society would like to give you access to our Cross Training exclusive bonus content.

You're only a click away from receiving:

The ultimate pre-workout ritual I use to smash my personal records

A guide detailing the only Cross Training equipment you should use while training

Exclusive pre-release access to our latest eBooks

Free Shredded Society eBooks during promotional periods

Simply navigate to:

http://shredded-society.com/WOD.html

in order to receive this bonus content

As this is a limited time offer it would be a shame to miss out, I recommend grabbing these bonuses before reading on.

Introduction

I would like to thank you and congratulate you for purchasing the book, *Bodyweight Cross Training WOD Bible: 220 Travel Friendly Home Workouts*

This book will introduce you to the many health & fitness benefits of the bodyweight training, along with 220 bodyweight WODs (workouts) you can implement immediately to improve your speed, strength and agility.

Thanks again for purchasing this book, I hope you enjoy it!

Benefits of Cross Training

Cross Training is not just a new fad amongst all the other styles of training that come and go throughout the years; Cross Training has many benefits these include:

Intensity

Cross Training workouts are fast paced and intense (as the emphasis is on speed and total weight being lifted), they are generally much shorter than a regular weight lifting workout – however since the workout is condensed it is constant non-stop movement, there is no time to stop and talk to your gym partner between sets like you normally would as you are constantly working against the clock to better yourself.

Creates Athletes

Cross Training exercises are all high power functional movements, this is highly emphasised. Cross Training, unlike bodybuilding does not believe in low power isolation movements. The major benefit here is now that the focus has been taken off vanity and looks it has been put 100% on performance – the core strength, stamina, coordination, agility and balance you will develop through participation in Cross Training will transfer over to sports and all other facets of life.

Time

The number one excuse for individuals not following a workout regime is the constraint of time; yes its true – working out takes time. However, Cross Training WODs are short - with many intense workouts ranging from 15 – 20 minutes they are faster and more effective than a regular workout in which you spend an hour on a cross trainer mindlessly staring at the wall.

Measureable Results

Cross Training workouts provide you with measureable and repeatable data; this can be used to verify that your fitness level is increasing. With a series of 'bench mark' workouts known as 'The Girls' and 'The Heroes' you can easily assess your progress.

Life Changing

Change your body, change your life, and change your world...
Cross Training workouts build mental strength, grit and confidence; a tough Cross Training workout will emotionally push you beyond your limits. When you ignore the voice inside your head that says 'it's too hard' or 'I can't do that last rep' and push past it unbreakable confidence is built – then anything is possible.

Community

Cross Training encourages community, both in the gym and online. People encourage and support each other through out their workouts – you will never have to work out alone again unless you want to, as the bond formed between training partners make training truly fun. It is very rarely you will find an individual that is as passionate about a particular pastime as yourself however this could not be further from the truth with the Cross Training community; we are all teammates that push and pray for each other.

Terminology

The following Cross Training terminology guide will come in helpful when interpreting your Cross Training workouts.

1RM: Your 1RM is your max lift for one rep

AHAP: as heavy as possible

AMRAP: As many rounds as possible

ATG: Ass to Grass

BP: Bench press

Box: Another name for a gym

BS: Back squat

BW: Body weight

CTT: Cross Training Total - consisting of max squat, press, and deadlift

CTWU: Cross Training Warm-up

Chipper: A WOD containing many different exercises and reps

CLN: Clean

C&J: Clean and jerk

C2: Concept II rowing machine

DL: Deadlift

DOMS: Delayed onset muscle soreness

DU: Double under

EMOM: Every minute on the minute

For Time: Timed workout, perform as quickly as possible and record score.

FS: Front squat

GHR(D): Glute ham raise (developer). Posterior chain exercise, similar to a back extension. Also, the device that allows for the proper performance of a Glute Ham Raise.

GHR(D) Situp: Situp performed on the GHR(D) bench.

GPP: General physical preparedness, another word for fitness

GTG: Grease the Groove, a protocol of doing many sub-maximal sets of an exercise throughout the day

H2H: Hand to hand; refers to Jeff Martone's kettlebell "juggling" techniques

HSPU: Hand stand push up. Kick up into a handstand (use wall for balance, if needed) bend arms until nose touches floor and push back up.

HSQ: Hang squat (clean or snatch). Start with bar "at the hang," about knee height. Initiate pull. As the bar rises drop into a full squat and catch the bar in the racked position. From there, rise to a standing position

IF: Intermittent Fasting

KB: Kettlebell

KBS: Kettlebell swing

KTE: Knees to elbows.

MetCon: Metabolic Conditioning workout

MP: Military press

MU: Muscle ups. Hanging from rings you do a combination pull-up and dip so you end in an upright support.

OH: Overhead

OHS: Overhead squat. Full-depth squat performed while arms are locked out in a wide grip press position above (and usually behind) the head.

PC: Power clean

Pd: Pood, weight measure for kettlebells

PR: Personal record

PP: Push press

PSN: Power snatch

PU: Pull-ups or push ups depending on the context in WOD

Rep: Repetition. One performance of an exercise.

RM: Repetition maximum.

ROM: Range of motion.

Rx'd: As prescribed, without any adjustments.

SDHP: Sumo deadlift high pull

Set: A number of repetitions. e.g., 34sets of 8 reps, often seen as 4x8, means you do 8 reps, rest, repeat, rest, repeat, rest, repeat.

SPP: Specific physical preparedness, aka skill training.

SN: Snatch

SQ: Squat

SS: Starting Strength; Mark Rippetoe's great book on strength training basics

Subbed: Substituted

T2B: Toes to bar. Hang from bar. Bending only at waist raise your toes to touch the bar, slowly lower them and repeat.

Tabata: A form of interval training comprised of 20 seconds on, 10 seconds off repeated for 8 rounds.

TGU: Turkish get-up

The Girls: A series of benchmark workouts named after girls

The Heroes: Brutal benchmark workouts in honour of fallen soldiers

TnG: Touch and go, no pausing between reps

WO: Workout

WOD: Workout of the day

YBF: You'll Be Fine

What is Bodyweight Training

Back in the day before adjustable dumbbells, magical weight loss pills, potions and all the 'fluff' that has riddled the fitness industry the individuals who set out to become strong, muscular and athletic relied on bodyweight based training… in these times it was performed as it was the only option – today it is still used because of how effective it is.

If we follow back the origins of bodyweight training the Spartans and romans both embraced bodyweight training, with the military and Navy SEALs constantly incorporating bodyweight based exercises in their training regimes and fitness tests.

This may partially be due to the convenience and minimal cost involved in performing these exercises, although there is no denying just how effective they are – regardless of any skills you may have, your currently fitness level or whether you are a fresh recruit as opposed to an army ranger a bodyweight workout regime will both challenge and improve wherever you currently are.

Outside of being used by ancient warriors and the modern day military bodyweight exercises play a large role in the training regimes of athletes around the world due to the immense fat loss and muscle gaining properties of this training.

Bodyweight exercises are known as Closed Kinetic Chain Exercises, without getting too technical this essentially means that either your hands or feet are in a constant held position (examples are squats, push ups, pullups, lunges). These Closed Kinetic Chain Exercises involve the use of multiple muscle groups and joints at once – a prime example of this is the bodyweight squat, during this exercise you are engaging your quads, hamstrings, glutes, calves and hip flexors.

On the other hand we have Open Chain Kinetic Exercises, an exercise is classed as OCK if the hand or foot of the individual performing the exercise is free to move throughout the exercise. Open Chain exercises isolate individual muscle groups and joints (think bicep curls or leg extensions). These exercises will induce hypertrophy, resulting in muscle gain although they are nowhere near as functional or safe as the CKC (bodyweight) style of training.

Closed Kinetic Chain Exercises essentially 'copy' activities that we all perform on a daily basis so unlike isolation style bodybuilding training it is a very functional form of training.

Now, let's have a look at the benefits of bodyweight training in a bit more detail.

Benefits of Bodyweight Training

Ultimate Efficiency:

Unless you're looking to become a professional bodybuilder or athlete there is simply no need to exercise for in excess of 2 hours with multiple apparatuses. An efficient workout regime comprising of high output bodyweight based exercises such as plyometrics and strength based exercise which require minimal set up and rest time between each other will provide you with the most efficient workout possible.

Cardio & Strength in One:

Bodyweight exercises such as burpees and push ups combine strength based training with cardiovascular endurance, you will burn calories while promoting muscle growth at the same time, no need to split your cardio and resistance workouts.

Torching the Fat:

Performing an intense bodyweight circuit comprising of exercises such as burpees, jumping jacks and sit-ups is guaranteed to get your metabolism firing, resulting in increased fat loss in a reduced period of time.

Universally Suitable:

The fantastic part apart bodyweight training is that it is entirely scalable, hence why the majority of personal trainers include bodyweight exercises in their boot camps and training sessions. Not everyone can do a squat below parallel or perform an overhead press correctly but everyone can perform a variation of the push up, whether this be on their toes, knees, wide hand placement or narrow hand placement.

Bodyweight exercises don't lie as progress is easy to gauge as you progress over time.

Flexibility:

Heavy, frequent resistance training can lead to inflexible or damaged joints and tight, non-functional muscles. If instead you perform bodyweight exercises to increase your strength while utilising a full range of motion on your exercises your joints will be permitted to move freely, you will also be reducing your risk of exercise related injury and will improve your posture over time. Bodyweight exercises are king for improving flexibility – Yoga is a prime example.

No Time, No Worries:

We all know the most common excuses for not exercising are a lack of time, no access to a gym or monetary issues. Well, all of these issues are alleviated with bodyweight training. A bodyweight exercise regime can be performed when you have 10 – 15 minutes of free time in a park, at home or even during your lunch break at work, since you're primarily lifting your bodyweight no expensive equipment is required!

Balance:

Overall awareness and control of your body will be increased through bodyweight training. Once you have mastered the basic exercises such as the bodyweight squat it's time to take it up a notch to single legged squats (referred to as a pistol squat) exercises like these will improve your overall balance, bodily awareness and athleticism.

Fun:

Following a gruelling workout regime in the confines of an old gym is not everyone's idea of enjoyable, bodyweight workouts are the polar opposite of this, you can assemble a group of friends and head outdoors for a bodyweight circuit, you'll get fit, fresh air and a laugh all at the same time.

Budget:

As mentioned briefly earlier, bodyweight training certainly does not break the bank. You can get in many solid workouts without any equipment at all, the only piece of equipment I tend to incorporate in my own bodyweight routines are a door way chin up bar and a skipping rope, together these cost me a grand total of $40 USD.
You do not need any money at all to begin bodyweight training.

Safe:

Heavy resistance exercise, if performed incorrectly can cause serious injury – damaged rotator cuffs, hernias and damaged discs are all too common today, these injuries all require a lengthy recovery and rehabilitation approach.
Bodyweight exercises are commonly used for rehabilitation, if you're looking to avoid aches and pains then bodyweight train should most certainly become a part of your exercise regime regardless of your age, gender or current fitness level.

Results:

Bodyweight training has been around since the beginning of fitness, it's not a new fad like many of the workout regimes that come and go each week on the news and in your local fitness magazines. Bodyweight regimes are comprised of compound exercises, meaning that multiple muscle groups and joints are utilised with each exercise. Compound exercises have been proven to be the most effective form of exercise for increased strength, size and athletic performance.

Bodyweight Training Principles

Become the master of your body

Before you decide to focus on how much you can deadlift or squat it is wise to learn to control and master the movement of your own bodyweight first.

Progressive overload applies

Just like lifting a barbell or pair of dumbbells, if you want to grow you need to progress, whether this be additional repetitions or a more advanced variation of the same exercise.

Abandon your comfort zone

Everyone has exercises they are not particularly good at or fond of, focus on these, commit to these otherwise you will begin to encounter imbalances which will stunt your progress lower down the line.

Experiment

Everyone is different; don't buy into the hype of certain exercises, routines or movements. Try everything to determine what works best for you.

Have fun with it

If you don't enjoy it you won't continue to do it. Make sure you're alternating your routine and exercises from time to time to ensure you're having fun while moving forward.

Focus on the function

Don't focus on the size of your biceps, focus on your ability to manoeuvre and lift your own bodyweight first, the aesthetics will come.

Don't rush

Don't expect instant results; learn to love the journey and slow, steady progression.
Going all out from day 1 can lead to tendon, ligament and connective tissue damage – fitness is a marathon not a sprint.

Fitness cannot be purchased

Fitness is one of few things in the world that cannot be purchased, you have to constantly work and strive for it.

Ratios

Your power to weight ratio is king, this ratio will give you a competitive advantage in sports and many other activities throughout life.

Work with what you have

Are you training in a park today? We'll you're lucky because that means you'll have access to a tree, several park benches and a set of stairs… work with what you have, it certainly doesn't need to be fancy.

Common Bodyweight Exercises

The following bodyweight exercises are the foundation of bodyweight training, each of these exercises is entirely scalable, and if performed correctly will transform your physique.

Squats

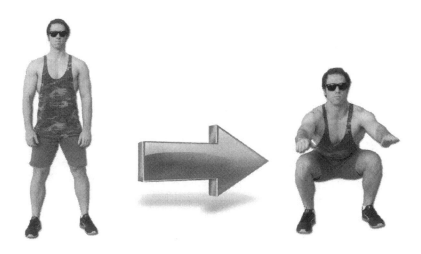

Description:

Squats are the ultimate lower body exercise - squats target the quads, glutes, hamstrings and core.

Form:

Begin with your feet shoulder width apart, place your hands wherever you find them most comfortable (by your sides, behind your head, in front of you).
Flex your hips and knees while sitting back, aim for your thighs to reach an angle parallel to the floor.
Reverse the movement to return to the starting position.

<u>Scaling</u>:

Beginners are to squat as deep as their body allows – the majority of individuals will not be able to get anywhere near parallel with correct form when starting.

Intermediate individuals are to ensure each repetition is to at least parallel.

Advanced are to perform ATG squat repetitions (ass to grass) meaning they will be below parallel on each and every repetition.

Push Ups

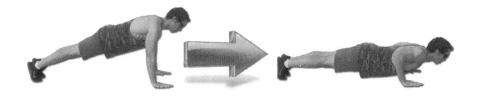

Description:

Push ups are by far the most common and popular bodyweight exercise.
Push ups work the chest, triceps and shoulders.

Form:

To perform a push up begin with your hands slightly wider than
shoulder width apart. Support your body on your toes as if you were
holding a plank position.
Keep your body as straight as possible.
Lower your chest to the ground by flexing your elbow joints.
Extend your elbows as your draw power through your pectoral muscles
to return to the starting position.

Scaling:

Beginners are to start on their knees as opposed to toes until they are
able to comfortably support their whole bodyweight.

Advanced athletes can perform push ups with their feet on a decline bench to allow a greater range of motion, or alternatively performed regular push up with additional weight e.g. a loaded backpack, weight vest or plate seated on their back.

Burpees

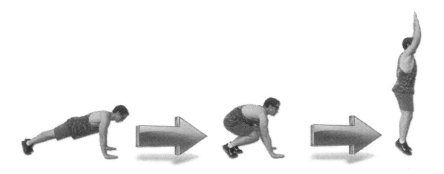

Description:

Burpees are designed to work your entire body with each and every repetition. Burpees will develop and test both your strength and aerobic based fitness, they're a quick and effective workout themselves!

Form:

Start in a squat position with your hands out infront of you.
Kick your feet backwards to assume a push up position.
Jump your feet forward to the initial squat position.
From the squat position jump as high as possible while raising your hands over head.

Scaling:

Beginners are to rest for 1 second between repetitions if necessary.

Intermediates are to perform consistent rep by rep without a rest period between.

Advanced are to perform a pull up upon completion of each rep (jump onto a pull up bar during the last squat jump portion of each repetition).

Tuck Jumps

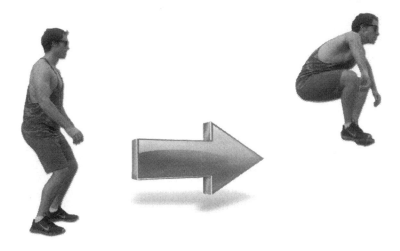

Description:

The tuck jump is fantastic for improving leg strength and explosive power – you'll develop your hamstrings and calves, if you play a sport such as basketball tuck jumps would be quite familiar.

Form:

Begin standing with knees slightly belt, hold your hands infront of you. Dip down to perform a partial squat before exploding upwards to drive your knees to your chest.
Re-extend your legs during each rep to absorb the landing and avoid injury.

Scaling:

Beginners are to rest for 1 second between repetitions if necessary.

Intermediates are to perform consistent rep by rep without a rest period between.

Pull Ups

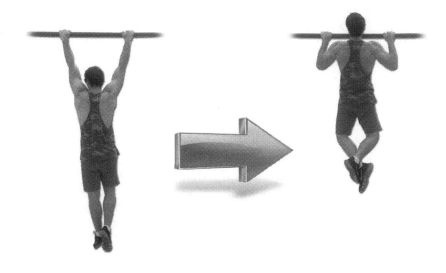

Description:

Pull ups are without a doubt the ultimate upper body bodyweight exercise, Red Bull won't give you wings, pull ups will! This exercise targets the lats and middle back with the biceps assisting as the secondary muscle group.

Form:

Using a wider than shoulder width grip, grasp the pullup bar with palms facing away from you.
Push your chest forward and curve your lower back slightly backwards to create a slight angle in your positioning.
Pull your body up by driving your shoulder blades and arms down/back – you want to be pulling through your back, not your biceps.
Hold for 1 second at the top of the rep with your chest touching the pullup bar.

32

Slowly lower yourself down until your arms are straight and fully extended.

<u>Scaling:</u>

Pull ups are by far one of the hardest bodyweight exercises to perform, not to worry though as they are highly scalable regardless of your current fitness and strength level.

Beginners are to perform the negative portion of the pull up in order to strengthen their back to gain the necessary strength to perform the full repetition, to do this – jump up and hold onto the pull up bar and slowly lower yourself down, the negative portion of the repetition should be slow and controlled, aim for a 3 – 5 second negative for each repetition.

Intermediates athletes are to perform the standard pull ups, ensuring their arms are fully extended to a dead hang at the end of each repetition.

Advanced athletes (those who can comfortably perform more than 10 repetitions per set) are to add a weighted vest, backpack or weighted belt to add additional resistance.

Box Jumps

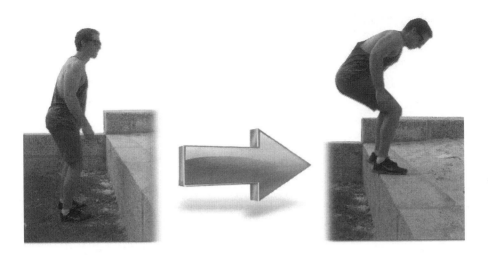

Description:

Box jumps are a fantastic plyometric exercise, box jumps will primarily build explosive strength and power in your hamstrings, with the quads, glutes, abductors and calves assisting as secondary muscles.

Form:

Start with your feet shoulder width apart in front of a box.
Drop your hips and flex your knees slightly to drop down into a partial squat, swing your arms behind you as you do so.
Extend explosively upwards by extending your hips, knees and ankles to jump upwards – use your arms for momentum.
Bend your knees slightly as you land on top of the box to soften the impact.

Swiftly jump back down to the ground.

Scaling:

Beginners are to start on a low box, and step down one leg at a time as opposed to jumping back down to complete the repetition.

Intermediate athletes are to perform the standard box jump, jumping both onto and back down from a moderate sized box.

Advanced athletes are to use a high box, jumping both onto and back down from the box.

Walking Lunges

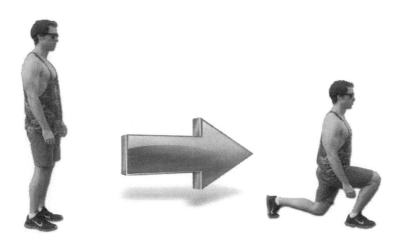

Description:

Walking lunges are a lower body compound exercise, lunges primarily target the quads, with hamstrings, glutes and calves acting as secondary muscles throughout the movement.

Form:

Start with a shoulder width stance with your hands placed on your hips. As you place one foot forward flex your knees in orer to drop your hips back, lower yourself until your rear knee brushes the ground.
Ensure your front foot is in line with your knee, maintain a straight back for the duration of the repetition.
Drive through the heel of your leading foot as you flex both knees to return to an upright position.
Repeat the above steps as you bring your rear foot forward.

<u>Scaling:</u>

Beginners are to perform walking lunges with small steps, placing emphasis on the quads.

Intermediate athletes are to take large steps enabling greater hamstring and glute activation (you will find these are substantially harder).

Advanced individuals are to hold a dumbbell or kettlebell in each hand as they perform their lunges for added resistance, do not allow the weights to touch the ground at all for the duration of your set.

Hand Stand Push Ups

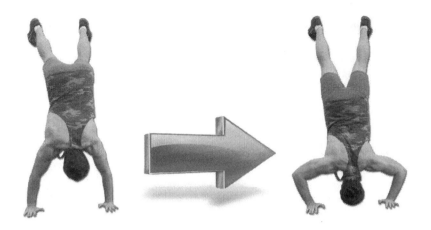

Description:

In my opinion the handstand push up, commonly referred to as HSPU is one of the most affective exercises to increase shoulder size and strength. The traditional handstand push up is quite an advanced exercise – however don't fret as there are several beginner and intermediate versions available that will have you performing the traditional HSPU in no time!

Form:

Place your hands shoulder width apart as you bend down against a wall. While maintaining straight arms kick yourself up against a wall. Position yourself against the wall with your arms and legs at a full extension, keep your body as straight as possible (tip: look at the wall, don't look down at the floor).
Lower yourself slowly until your head almost touches the ground.
Push yourself up until your arms are fully extended (locked out).

Scaling:

Beginners are to progressively build up to the hand stand push up by performing regular push ups with their feet elevated on a small stool or bench, the higher the incline the more stress you will be placing on your shoulders. Slowly work your way up to higher objects such as a stool, bench or table.

Intermediate individuals are to perform regular hand stand push ups against a wall.

Once you can comfortably perform a number of repetitions of the traditional hand stand push up against a wall it's time to take it to the next level – the free standing hand stand push up.
Perform a hand stand and maintain your balance as you begin to perform your push ups, you will require a high level of balance and core strength to perform this advanced variation.

Dips

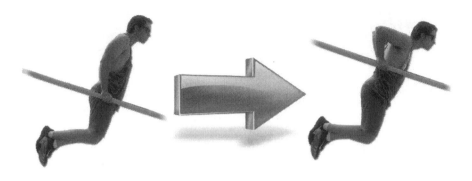

Description:

Dips are a great upper body compound exercise that can be performed in 2 different variations based upon whether you would like to place greater emphasis on the chest or the triceps. Your anterior deltoids (front of your shoulders) are also targeted as a secondary muscle group as you perform dips.

Form:

Tricep Dip:

Assume an arm's length position from your parallel bars with arms locked out.
While maintaining an upright position with elbows closed to your position begin to lower your body until your upper arm and forearm resemble a 90 degree angle.
Push through your triceps to bring yourself back to the starting position.

Chest Dip:

Assume an arm's length position from your parallel bars with arms locked out.
Begin to lower yourself with your elbows flared out and your body leaned forward at roughly a 30 degree angle.
Lower yourself until you begin to feel a deep stretch in your chest.
Use your chest to push your body back up to the starting position, ensuring you maintain the 30 degree angle throughout the exercise.

Scaling:

Beginners are to perform bent knee bench dips.
In order to do this place your hands on a bench or chair that is behind you, begin to lower yourself until your backside touches the floor.
Breathe out as you push yourself back up.
Once the bent knee bench dip has been mastered proceed to place your legs on another chair or bench, ensuring they are straight and raised – allowing you to lift a greater portion of your bodyweight.

Intermediate individuals are to perform the standard bodyweight dips, ensuring a full range of motion is being utilised.

Advanced individuals (those whom are able to perform 12+ bodyweight dips comfortably) are to add resistance with either a weight belt, weighted vest or by placing a dumbbell between your legs.

Double Unders

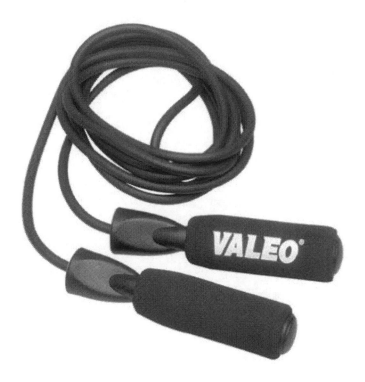

Description:

Skipping is a great tool for conditioning, Rocky and Muhammad Ali are great examples of those whom embraced skipping for their fitness. The double under is a skipping exercise in which the skipping rope passes underneath your feet twice while you perform one slightly higher than normal jump. This requires skill, timing and coordination to pull off successfully.

Form:

Perform several single unders to warm up and get into the correct timing before attempting the double under.

Jump higher than usual, as you do swing the rope for 2 full revolutions, you do not need to extend your arms like windmills – it is all in the wrist.

Land and continue to skip/perform double unders.

Scaling:

Beginners are to alternate between single unders and double unders

Advanced individuals are to perform continuous double unders with no rest or single unders between repetitions.

Pistol Squat

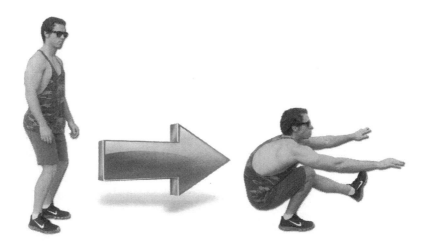

Description:

The pistol squat will test and increase your flexibility and balance while primarily working your quads with the hamstrings, glutes and calves acting as secondary muscle groups. This exercise is highly scalable as beginners will unlikely be able to initially perform a full depth pistol squat.

Form:

Hold your arms out in front of your to assist with balance.
Hold one of your legs off of the floor and begin to squat down on the other leg by flexing your knee and driving your hips backwards.
Drive through your heel to return to the upright position, keep your head and chest up for the duration of the exercise.

Scaling:

Beginners are to perform the pistol squat while holding onto a rail or bench with one arm, this will allow you to gain flexibility and familiarise yourself with the squatting motion without having to stabilise yourself completely.

Intermediate individuals are to perform pistol squats onto a low bench or seat, this will allow you to have a brief pause at the bottom portion of each repetition to take the stress temporarily off the quads and allowing you to regain balance if necessary.

Advanced individuals are to perform the regular pistol squat while grasping onto a kettlebell or dumbbell with both hands.

Sit-up

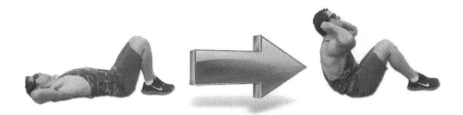

Description:

The sit-up is the most common abdominal exercise in existence, sit-ups are performed to increase core strength. It is worth noting that you will not get six pack abdominals simply by performing sit-ups or any other abdominal exercise for that matter, this comes down to a manipulation of diet to achieve single digit body fat – at which time your abdominal region will be visible.

Form:

Lay on the floor with your feet hooked under a bench or object to prevent movement.
Interlock your hands behind your head.
Elevate your shoulders and upper back off the ground by engaging your abdominal muscles.
Breathe out as you contract your abdominals.
Lower yourself back down slowly while breathing in.

<u>Scaling:</u>

Beginners are to perform regular sit-ups on a flat surface.

Intermediate individuals are to perform sit-ups on a decline bench or similar to allow for a greater range of motion.

Advanced individuals can perform decline sit-ups while holding a dumbbell or weight plate for additional resistance.

Plank

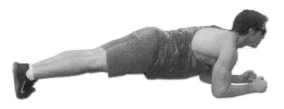

Description:

A simple exercise that yields massive results.
The plank is a static hold in which the abdominal muscles are used to
stabilise the body.

Form:

Assume a prone position with your weight being held by your forearms
and toes, keep your forearms directly below your shoulders.
Hold this position while maintaining a straight body for the duration of
the plank.

Scaling:

Beginners are to perform the standard plank for 30 second per plank.

Intermediate individuals are to perform a plank for 45 seconds while
raising either 1 arm or 1 leg off the ground for the duration of the
plank.

Advanced individuals are to perform a plank for 1 minute while raising
1 arm and the opposite leg off the ground for the duration of the
plank.

Side Plank

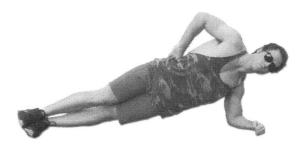

Description:

The side plank is a great exercise for tightening the intricate portions of the abdominal region, specifically the obliques and transverse abdominus. Lower back strength is also significantly increased which will reduce your risk of certain lower back injuries.

Form:

To perform the side plank lie on one side with your knees straight forward.
Support your upper body with your elbow and forearm, your elbow should be positioned under your shoulder.
Tighten your core and raise your hips so your body forms a straight line all the way from your ankles to your shoulders.
Hold the side plank for the prescribed duration.
Repeat above steps for the opposite side.

Scaling:

Beginners are to perform the side plank on bent knees as opposed to toes, this will decrease the portion of your body weight you are supporting.

Intermediate individuals are to perform the standard side plank for a duration of 30 seconds.

Advanced individuals are to alternate between the standard side plank, supporting your body with your elbow to straight arm planks, supporting your body with your hand – arm fully extended.

Mountain Climbers

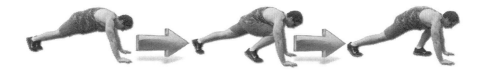

Description:

Mountain climbers are a great plyometric style of exercise that will get your heart pumping! Mountain climbers work the quads as the primary muscle group, with some chest, hamstrings and shoulders also coming in to play.

Form:

Start in a push-up position; support your bodyweight on your hands and toes.
Flex your knee and hip to bring one leg forward and upwards until the knee is underneath your hip, this is where we'll start the exercise.
Reverse the position of your leg by extending the bent leg until it is straight, bring your other foot forward by flexing your knee and hip.
Continue to alternate for the desired number of repetitions.

Scaling:

Beginners and intermediate individuals are to perform standard mountain climbers as described.

Advanced individuals are to bring your knees to the side of your body, as opposed to directly in front of you, these are substantially harden and are often referred to as side to side climbers.

Bodyweight WODs

On the following pages you will find 220 bodyweight based workouts, these workouts can be performed anywhere and are designed to burn fat and build muscle without occupying a large portion of your day.

WOD 1
3 rounds for time:
10 burpees
20 squats
30 situps

WOD 2
tabata (8 intervals – 20 seconds work – 10 seconds rest):
Pushups
Situps
Squats

WOD 3
5 rounds for time:
10 tuck jumps
15 back extensions

WOD 4
2 rounds for time:
400m run
50 lunges

WOD 5
For time:
100 pushups
50 situps

WOD 6
3 rounds for time:

20 burpees
30 squats
40 situps

WOD 7
4 rounds for time:
15 tuck jumps
25 situps

WOD 8
For time:
100 burpees

WOD 9
5 rounds for time:
20 burpees
10 situps
20 squats

WOD 10
For time:
5km run

WOD 11
For time:
50 box jumps

50 walking lunges
20 burpees

WOD 12
5 rounds for time:
20 jumping squats
20 sit ups
20 push ups

WOD 13
For time:
500m row
50 squats
40 sit ups
30 push ups
10 burpees

WOD 14
AMRAP
1 minute plank
15 bicycle crunches
10 burpees
1 minute plank
15 bicycle crunches
20 squats

WOD 15
3 rounds for time:
10 push ups
20 squats
10 crunches

10 burpees
25 jumping jacks
20 second plank
20 lunges

WOD 16
3 rounds for time:
200m sprint
15 pushups
15 lunges
100m sprint
15 squats

WOD 17
5 rounds for time:
15 push ups
15 sit ups
15 jump squats

WOD 18
1 minute plank
500 meter run
2 minute plank
500 meter run
3 minute plank
500m cool down jog

WOD 19
4 rounds for time:
20 walking lunges
20 push ups
20 jumping jacks

WOD 20
AMRAP
20 squats
100 meter run
20 walking lunges
10 push ups
10 lunges
100 meter run

WOD 21
3 rounds for time:
15 vertical jumps
15 jumping jacks
10 burpees
15 push ups

WOD 22
1 round for time:
skip for 1 minute
20 vertical jumps
20 jumping jacks
skip for 1 minute
20 squats
20 walking lunges

WOD 23
AMRAP
20 sit ups
20 reverse crunches
20 high knees
20 squat jumps
10 pushups

WOD 24
7 rounds for time:
7 burpees
7 squats
7 sit ups
7 jumping jacks

WOD 25
3 rounds for time:
90 second plank
20 burpees
90 second plank
20 vertical jumps

WOD 26
Walking lunges for 400m

WOD 27
150 burpees

WOD 28
4 rounds of:
Run 400m
50 squats
100-75-50-25 reps:
situps
flutterkicks
Leg levers

WOD 29
50 burpees

WOD 30
Cumulative L-hold for 5 minutes
Use a bar, rings, or floor

WOD 31
50 squats
25 pushups
50 pistol squats
25 fingertip pushups
50 side lunges
25 knuckle pushups
50 walking lunges
25 diamond pushups

WOD 32

50 flutterkicks
50 situps
Run 400m
100 flutterkicks
100 situps
Run 400m

WOD 33
20-16-12-8-4 reps of:
One-arm pushups
Pistol squats

WOD 34
4 rounds of:
50 pushups
50 situps
50 flutterkicks

WOD 35
1 round Tabata sprints (8 rounds, 20 seconds on, 10 seconds off)
1 round Tabata bottom-to-bottom squats (8 rounds, 20 seconds on, 10 seconds off)

WOD 36
AMRAP in 12 minutes of:
10 pushups
15 situps
20m walking lunge

WOD 37
21-15-9 reps of:
lunges
situps
burpees

WOD 38
5 rounds of:
50 mountain climbers
25 situps

WOD 39
5 rounds of:
100 jumping jacks
100 mountain climbers

WOD 39
Burpees: 20-19-18-17 ...4- 3-2-1
Walk 25m after each set

WOD 40
50 rounds of:
1 squat
1 pushup
1 situp
1 superman
1 tuck jump

WOD 41
50 jumping jacks
50 pushups
50 tuck jumps
50 situps
50 mountain climbers
50 squats
50 jumping jacks

WOD 42
10 rounds:
30 second handstand

30 second isometric squat

WOD 43
Run 100m
20 pushups
5 burpees
15 clap pushups
5 burpees
10 chest-slap pushups
5 burpees
5 fingertip pushups
Run 100m
15 pushups
5 burpees
10 clap pushups
5 burpees
10 chest-slap pushups
5 burpees
5 fingertip pushups
Run 100m
10 pushups
5 burpees
10 clap pushups

WOD 44
5 burpees
10 chest-slap pushups
5 burpees
5 fingertip pushups

WOD 45
Run 400m
Burpee-Broad Jump 25m
Walking Lunges 25m
Burpee-Broad Jump 25m
Bear Crawl 25m
Burpee-Broad Jump 25m

Walking Lunges 25m
Burpee-Broad Jump 25m
Bear Crawl 25m
Run 400m

WOD 46
100 situps
100 flutterkicks
100 leg levers

WOD47
Use a deck of cards:
Face cards= 10
Aces = 11
Numbered cards are as per number states
Flip each card and perform the movement and the number of reps specified
WOD is complete once the whole deck has been utilised
Hearts - burpees
Diamonds – mountain climbers
Spades - flutterkicks
Clubs - situps
Jokers - Run 400m

WOD 48
50 burpees
75 flutterkicks
100 pushups
150 situps

WOD 49
5 rounds:
10 burpees
20 box jumps
30 pushups
40 squats
50 lunges

WOD 50
4 rounds:
50 walking lunges
50 squats
Run 400m

WOD 51
Run 5km
Stop every 120 seconds to perform 20 pushups, 20 situps and 20 squats

WOD 52
3 rounds:
50 pushups
50 situps
50 squats

WOD 53
5 rounds:
50 walking lunges
15 handstand pushups
80 squats
10 handstand pushups
60 squats
20 handstand pushups
40 squats
30 handstand pushups
20 squats

WOD 54
4 rounds:

25 lunges
50 squats
5 rounds of:
100 squats
20 lunges
35 pushups

WOD 55
5 rounds of:
50 squats
30 handstand pushups

WOD 56
2 rounds:
Max pushups in 2 minutes
Max situps in 2 minutes
Max flutterkicks in 2 minutes
Max squats in 2 minutes

WOD 57
3 rounds of:
30 yard bear crawl
30 yard inch worm pushup
30 yard burpee jumps

WOD 58
100 burpee pullups

WOD 59
AMRAP in 20 minutes of:
15 pullups
30 pushups
45 squats

WOD 60

1 round:
Handstand pushups: 15-13-11-9-7-5-3-1
L-pullups: 1-3-5-7-9-11-13-15

WOD 61
3 rounds:
Run 800m
50 pullups

WOD 62
10 rounds:
12 burpees
12 pullups

WOD 63
5 rounds:
15 L-pullups
30 pushups
45 situps

WOD 64
5 rounds:
25 inverted burpees
25 pullups
25 burpees

WOD 65
30 handstand pushups
10 pullups
20 handstand pushups
20 pullups
10 handstand pushups
30 pullups

WOD 66

Run 800m
40 L-pullups
Run 800m
40 strict pullups
Run 800m
40 kipping pullups

WOD 67
5 rounds of:
50 squats
30 pullups
15 handstand pushups
100 squats
100 pullups
200 pushups
300 squats
100 lunges

WOD 68
21-15-9 reps of:
burpees
pullups

WOD 69
21-15-9 reps of:
pullups
pushups
squat jumps to 14" above max reach

WOD 70
50-35-20 rep rounds of:
handstand pushups
pullups

WOD 71

AMRAP in 15 minutes:
20 seconds of pullups
20 seconds of situps
20 seconds of squats

WOD 72
100 pullups
200 pushups
300 squats
50 situps

WOD 73
AMRAP in 20 minutes of:
25 pullups
50 pushups
75 squats

WOD 74
AMRAP in 20 minutes of:
25 handstand pushups
50 pistol squats
75 pullups

WOD 75
AMRAP in 20 minutes of:
10 L pullups
20 squats

WOD 76
Run 1600M
100 bodyblasters (burpee-pullups-knees to elbows)
Run 1600M

WOD 77
Tabata pullups, 1 round
Run 1600m
Tabata pushups, 1 round
Run 1600m
Tabata situps, 1 round

Run 1600m
Tabata squats, 1 round
Run 1600m

WOD 78
10-20-30 reps of:
squat
handstand pushups
squat
pullups

WOD 79
100 pullups
Run 1 mile
100 pushups
Run 1 mile
100 situps
Run 1 mile
100 squats
Run 1 mile

WOD 80
Run 1 mile
50 pullups
100 pushups
150 situps
200 squats
Run 1 mile
50 pullups
100 pushups
150 situps
200 squats
Run 1 mile

WOD 81
5 rounds of:

30 handstand pushups
30 pullups

WOD 82
100 squats
20 handstand pushups
30 pullups
100 squats
9 handstand pushups
200 squats
15 handstand pushups
100 squats
21 handstand pushups

WOD 83

100 L-pullups
100 squats
40 pullups
80 squats
32 pullups
60 squats
24 pullups
40 squats
16 pullups
20 squats
8 pullups

WOD 84

10 rounds of:
10 pullups
20 pushups
30 squats

WOD 85

AMRAP in 20 minutes of:
7 handstand pushups
12 L-pullups

WOD 86

50 squats
50 pullups
50 walking lunges
50 knees-to-elbows
5 handstand pushups
50 situps
5 handstand pushups
50 squats
50 pullups

WOD 87
100 squats
25 situps
100 squats
25 situps
100 squats
25 knees-to-elbows
100 squats
25 handstand pushups

WOD 88
2 rounds of:
35 squats
35 knees-to-elbows
35 squats
35 situps
35 lunges
35 squats

WOD 89
21-18-15-12-9-6-3 of:
squats
L-pullups
knees-to-elbows

WOD 90
7 rounds of:
35 squats
25 pushups
15 pullups

WOD 91
21-15-9 reps of:
Body blasters (burpee-pullup-knees to elbows)
box jump burpees

Belushi burpees (on jump turn 180 degrees)
Burpee Jacks (plank jack to jumping jack)

WOD 92
3 rounds of:
100 squats
25 L-pullups
30 handstand pushups
5 rounds of:
9 handstand pushups
9 pullups

WOD 93
21 pullups
50 squats
21 knees-to-elbows
18 pullups
50 squats
18 knees-to-elbows
15 pullups
50 squats
15 knees-to-elbows
12 pullups
50 squats
12 knees-to-elbows

WOD 94
20 rounds of:
5 pullups
5 pushups
5 situps
5 squats

WOD 95
100 squats

21 handstand pushups
30 pullups
100 squats
30 pullups
21 handstand pushups
100 squats

WOD 96
5 rounds of:
20 squats
20 pushups
20 pullups

WOD 97
50-40-30-20-10 reps
pullups
squat jumps

WOD 98
15 rounds for max reps:
Pullups - 30 seconds on 20 seconds off

WOD 99
100 squats
20 handstand pushups
30 pullups
100 squats
30 pullups
20 handstand pushups
100 squats

WOD 100
Run 400m
25 pullups
25 pushups

25 situps
25 squats

WOD 101
150 squats
50 pushups
21 pullups
Run 800m
21 pullups
50 pushups
150 squats

WOD 102
50 L-pullups
50 handstand pushups
50 pistol squats
50 knees-to-elbows

WOD 103
3 rounds of:
Run 800m
30 burpees
30 knees-to-elbows

WOD 104
21-15-9 reps of:
handstand pushups
Inverted pullups

WOD 105
20 Burpee Pullups
Run 800m
20 Burpee Pullups
Run 800m

20 Burpee Pullups

WOD 106
3 rounds:
10 push ups
10 jumping jacks
10 squats
10 jumping jacks
10 situps
10 jumping jacks

WOD 107
5 rounds:
20 sit-ups
30 second plank
15 sit-ups
30 second side plank (left)
15 sit-ups
30 second side plank (right)
10 sit-ups

WOD 108
3 rounds:
10 pullups
10 burpees
10 pullups
10 dips
10 burpees
10 dips
50 situps

WOD 109

2 rounds:
20 push-ups
20 squats
20 lunges (10 per leg)
20 sit-ups
200m run

WOD 110

4 rounds
10 double unders
20 single unders
200m run
5 burpees

WOD 111

4 rounds
10 jumping jacks
20 push-ups
30 sit-ups
3 planks

WOD 112

30 push-ups
10 HSPU
5 pull-ups
30 sit-ups
30 walking lunges (15 per leg)

WOD 113

3 rounds
50 squats

25 walking lunges
10 box jumps
5 burpees

WOD 114
5 rounds
100m sprint
30 push-ups
30 sit-ups
30 squats

WOD 115
1 round
1 pull-up
1 burpee
2 pull-ups
2 burpees
3 pull-ups
3 burpees
4 pull-ups
4 burpees
5 pull-ups
5 burpees
6 pull-ups
6 burpees
7 pull-ups
7 burpees
8 pull-ups
8 burpees
9 pull-ups
9 burpees
10 pull-ups

10 burpees

WOD 116
4 rounds
30 squats
30 walking lunges (15 per leg)
30 box jumps
10 burpees

WOD 117
5 rounds
20 pistol squats (10 per leg)
100m sprint
20 squats
100m sprint
20 walking lunges (10 per leg)
100m sprint

WOD 118
3 rounds
20 burpees
15 box jumps
10 push-ups
45 sit-ups

WOD 119
2 rounds
40 lunges (20 per leg)
10 dips
10 push-ups
10 HSPU
40 pistol squats (20 per leg)

WOD 120
3 rounds
20 double unders
50 push-ups
50 sit-ups
50 squats
20 double unders

WOD 121
4 rounds
20 side planks (left)
40 sit-ups
20 side planks (right)
20 box jumps
20 push-ups

WOD 122
1 round
100 single unders
50 jumping jacks
10 pull-ups
20 push-ups
30 sit-ups
40 squats

WOD 123
1 round
10 pull-ups
100m sprint
10 pull-ups
100m sprint

50 push-ups
500m jog

WOD 124
2 rounds
50 jumping jacks
50 mountain climbers
50 sit-ups

WOD 125
For time
100 pull-ups
100 HSPU

WOD 126
200 sit-ups
10 planks

WOD 127
for time
100 squats
50 walking lunges (25 per leg)
20 pistol squats (10 per leg)
100m sprint

WOD 128
for time
50 burpees
50 push-ups
50 sit-ups

WOD 129
2 rounds
50 squats
50 lunges (25 per leg)
50 mountain climbers

WOD 130
2 rounds
5 HSPU
10 push-ups
15 squats
20 walking lunges (10 per leg)
25 sit-ups

WOD 131
For time
200 pull-ups (break up into as many sets as necessary)
200 push-ups (break up into as many sets as necessary)

WOD 131
2 rounds
50m sprint
50 burpees
50m sprint
50 jumping jacks

WOD 132
1 round
100 squats
10 burpees
50 squats
20 burpees
10 sit-ups

WOD 133

2 rounds
20 tuck jumps
20 push ups
20 mountain climbers
50 walking lunges (25 per leg)

WOD 134

100 single unders
35 push ups
100 single unders
35 sit-ups
1 plank

WOD 135

2 rounds:
50 walking lunges (25 per leg)
50 seconds of single unders
50 squats
50 seconds of single unders
50 push-ups
50 seconds of single unders
50 sit-ups
50 seconds of single unders

WOD 136

10 rounds
1 pull-up
2 push-ups
3 squats
4 walking lunges (2 per leg)
5 mountain climbers

WOD 137

5 rounds
10 pull-ups
100m sprint

WOD 138

for time
200 air squats

WOD 140

25 push-ups
200m run
25 push-ups
50 jumping jacks

WOD 141

20 rounds for time
5 sit-ups
5 push-ups
5 squats

WOD 142

5 HSPU
5 air squats
5 push-ups
5 mountain climbers

WOD 143

10 rounds for time
100m sprint
100m walk

WOD 144
Tabata squats (20 seconds on 10 seconds off, 8 rounds)

WOD 145
3 rounds
20 jumping jacks
30 air squats
40 sit-ups

WOD 146
AMRAP in 15 minutes
10 push-ups
15 sit-ups
20 squats

WOD 147
Run 500m
50 squats
Run 500m
50 sit-ups

WOD 148
21-15-9
Push-ups
Bench dips
HSPU

WOD 149
For time
50 walking lunges (25 per leg)
1km run
50 walking lunges (25 per leg)

10 mountain climbers

WOD 150
10 rounds
10 burpees
50 jumping jacks

WOD 151
For time
50 squats
50 sit-ups
50 burpees
50 walking lunges (25 per leg)
50 push-ups

WOD 152
Accumulate 10 minutes in a handstand position

WOD 153
6 rounds
10 HSPU
15 push-ups
20 sit-ups

WOD 154

2 rounds
1 minute plank
1 minute rest
45 second plank
45 second rest
30 second plank
30 second rest

20 second plank
20 second rest
10 second plank
10 second rest

WOD 155
10 rounds
15 burpees
15 sit-ups

WOD 156
40 walking lunges (20 per leg)
30 sit-ups
20 supermans
15 push-ups

WOD 157
2 rounds
50 double unders
50 lunges (25 per leg)
50 sit-ups

WOD 158
Complete in 12 minutes
30 burpees
15 squats
20 burpees
30 squats
10 burpees
60 squats

WOD 159

4 rounds
20 bench dips
20 mountain climbers
20 pistol squats (10 per leg)

WOD 160

for time
100 burpees
20 squats
10 tuck jumps

WOD 161

20 seconds of high knees
20 seconds of push-ups
20 seconds rest
20 seconds of high knees
20 seconds of push-ups
20 seconds rest
20 seconds of high knees
20 seconds of push-ups
20 seconds rest
20 seconds of high knees
20 seconds of push-ups
20 seconds rest
20 seconds of high knees
20 seconds of push-ups

WOD 162

AMRAP in 20 minutes
15 push-ups
10 sit-ups
15 squats

WOD 163

40-30-15 of
burpees
push-up
jumping jack

WOD 164

4 rounds
30 second plank
10 push-ups
10 jumping jacks
10 mountain climbers

WOD 165

22 pistol squats (11 per leg)
6 HSPU
22 pistol squats (11 per leg)
6 HSPU
12 pistol squats (6 per leg)
3 HSPU

WOD 166

2 minutes max repetition push-ups
1 minute rest
2 minutes max repetition push-ups
1 minute rest
2 minutes max repetition push-ups
1 minute rest
2 minutes max repetition push-ups
1 minute rest
Bench dips until failure

WOD 167
500 jumping jacks
** stop after every 50 repetitions to perform 10 burpees **

WOD 168
3 rounds
50 squats
50 bench dips
30 second handstand

WOD 169
8 rounds
20 burpees
20 second handstand

WOD 170
6 rounds
15 jumping jacks
18 walking lunges (9 per leg)
15 push-ups
15 sit-ups
1 minute plank

WOD 171
AMRAP in 10 minutes
50 push-ups
50 sit-ups
50 squats

WOD 172
for time
400 walking lunges (200 per leg)

WOD 173
8 rounds
10 pistol squats (5 per leg)
1 minute plank
10 jumping jacks

WOD 174
3 rounds
5 clapping push-ups
10 supermans
30 walking lunges (15 per leg)

WOD 175
30 rounds
5 jumping jacks
2 burpees
3 push-ups

WOD 176
10 rounds
10 push-ups
100m sprint

WOD 177
4 rounds
10 sit-ups
10 burpees
10 walking lunges (5 per leg)

10 air squats

WOD 178
10 box jumps
50 sit-ups
50 air squats
400m run

WOD 179
7 rounds
20 seconds of mountain climbers
20 seconds of squats
20 seconds of pistol squats (each leg)

WOD 180
30 unbroken double unders
** as many attempts as necessary **

WOD 181
15 seconds of high knees
5 push-ups
15 seconds of high knees
5 push-ups
15 seconds of high knees
5 push-ups
15 seconds of high knees
5 push-ups
15 seconds of high knees
5 push-ups
15 seconds of high knees

5 push-ups
20 sit-ups
200m run

WOD 182

AMRAP in 12 minutes
3 burpees
6 supermans
9 sit-ups
12 push-ups

WOD 183
4 rounds
20 tuck jumps
10 push-ups
30 second handstand
20 walking lunges (10 per leg)
30 second plank

WOD 184
2 mile run for best time

WOD 185
Max distance in 30 minutes

WOD 186
1 round Tabata uphill sprints (20:10 x 8)

WOD 187
4 rounds of:
5:00 max distance
3:00 recovery

WOD 188
3 rounds:
5km run with 30 second recovery between rounds

WOD 189
1.2km uphill sprint
Rest 1:00
1.2km downhill jog
Rest 1:00
Repeat

WOD 190
1:00 sprint, 1:00 rest
1:00 sprint, 0:50 rest
1:00 sprint, 0:40 rest
1:00 sprint, 0:30 rest
1:00 sprint, 0:20 rest
1:00 sprint, 0:10 rest
1:00 sprint, 0:20 rest
1:00 sprint, 0:30 rest

1:00 sprint, 0:40 rest
1:00 sprint, 0:50 rest
1:00 sprint, 1:00 rest

WOD 191
10x100m with 2:00 rest
8x200m with 2:00 rest
4x400m with 5:00 rest
8 rounds of:
80 second sprint, 40 second rest

WOD 192
3 rounds of:
1:00 sprint, 1:00 recovery
2:00 sprint, 2:00 recovery
3:00 sprint, 3:00 recovery

WOD 193
3:00 sprint, 3:00 recovery
2:00 sprint, 2:00 recovery
1:00 sprint, 1:00 recovery
2:00 sprint, 2:00 recovery
3:00 sprint, 3:00 recovery

WOD 194
4x800m with 2:00 rest
Run 10k. Run second half faster than the first.

WOD 195
3 rounds of:
100m sprint, Rest same amount of time you finished the sprint
200m sprint, Rest same amount of time you finished the sprint
300m sprint, Rest same amount of time you finished the sprint

WOD 196

3 rounds of:
200m sprint, Rest same amount of time you finished the sprint
400m sprint, Rest same amount of time you finished the sprint
600m sprint, Rest same amount of time you finished the sprint

WOD 197
10 rounds of:
1:00 sprint, 1:00 recovery

WOD 198
8 rounds of:
10 seconds sprint, 5 seconds recovery

WOD 199
0:45 sprint, 0:45 recovery
1:30 sprint, 1:30 recovery
3:00 sprint, 3:00 recovery
6:00 sprint, 6:00 recovery
3:00 sprint, 3:00 recovery
1:30 sprint, 1:30 recovery
0:45 sprint, 0:45 recovery

WOD 200
16 rounds of:
10 seconds sprint, 20 seconds recovery

WOD 201
4x200m + 4x400m + 2x1000m
Rest 1:00, 1:30, and 2:00 per interval distance, respectively.

WOD 202
200m sprint, Rest same amount of time you finished the sprint
400m sprint, Rest same amount of time you finished the sprint
600m sprint, Rest same amount of time you finished the sprint

400m sprint, Rest same amount of time you finished the sprint
200m sprint, Rest same amount of time you finished the sprint

WOD 203
1 mile time trial
Rest 60 seconds
2x400m sprint
Rest 60 seconds between sprints

WOD 204
4x200m
2x400m
Rest 60 seconds between sprints

WOD 205
For time:
Run 3km
Row 3k
Run 1km

WOD 206
For time:
Cover a 1600m distance by performing burpees.
Perform a large jump with each rep.

WOD 207
3 rounds:
1 mile run
100 pullups,
200 pushups,
300 squats
1 mile run
First round to be completed with a weighted vest, partition as necessary
Second round is to be completed without partitions
Third round to be partitioned as necessary

WOD 208

500 pullups
500 pushups
500 situps
500 flutterkicks
500 squats
Partition as necessary

WOD 209

10 rounds of:
100 jump ropes
10 burpees
10 situps
10 pushups
10 squats
10 pullups

WOD 210

400m of burpees
400m walking lunges
400m bear crawl
400m reverse straight-legged bear crawl

WOD 211

Run 100m
50 burpees
Run 200m
100 pushups
Run 300m
150 walking lunges
Run 400m
200 squats
Run 300m
150 walking lunges
Run 200m
100 pushups

Run 100m
50 burpees

WOD 212
10 rounds of:
Max burpees 60 seconds
Max pullups 60 seconds
Max tuck jumps 60 seconds
Max jumping jacks 60 seconds
Max distance running 60 seconds

WOD 213
Station A: running
Station B: burpees
Station C: pullups
Station D: squat jumps
Station E: bear crawl or lunges
Round 1: 5:00 at each station, for total of 25:00.
Round 2: 12:00 at each station, for total of 1:00:00.
Round 3: 30:00 at each station, for total of 2:30:00.
Round 4: 1:00 at each station, for total of 5:00.

WOD 214
60 rounds of:
Run 400m
3 handstand pushups
2 pistols
1 muscle up

WOD 215

110 minutes: March with rucksack
15 minutes: Eat, hydrate, stretch, change clothes if necessary.
60 minutes: Run at half marathon pace.
60 minutes: Complete 1000 walking lunges.
30 minutes: 5 rounds: ring dips 1:00, rest 1:00, ring pushups 1:00, rest 1:00
60 minutes: Run at half marathon pace.
15 minutes: Eat, hydrate, stretch, change clothes if necessary.
30 minutes: Complete Angie, max intensity.
15 minutes: Sprint 10x100m with 1:00 rests.
15 minutes: Complete 100 burpees.
30 minutes: 4 rounds: 50 squats, 5 muscle ups. Sub 3/3 for MU if necessary.
30 minutes: 500 situps.
10 minutes: Run 1 mile.

WOD 216

Begin with 2 muscle ups, then 4 pistol squats + 2 muscleups, then 6 one-armed pushups + 4 pistol squats + 4 muscle ups, continuing to the rest of the workout at 30.

2 muscle-up
4 pistols
6 one-armed pushups
8 L-pullups
10 toes to bar
12 skin the cats
14 ring dips
16 5 foot broad jumps
18 pushups
20 air squats
22 box jumps
24 lunges
26 double unders
28 burpees
30 jingle-jangles

WOD 217

100 dead hang pull-ups
250 push-ups
500 sit-ups
Run 3 miles

WOD 218
For time
50 dead hang pull-ups
100 push-ups
150 sit-ups
200 squats

WOD 219
1 push-up
1 squat
2 push-ups
2 squats
3 push-ups
3 squats
4 push-ups
4 squats
Continue until failure

WOD 220
500m run
50 burpees
400m run
40 burpees
300m run
30 burpees
200m run
20 burpees
100m run
10 burpees

BONUS CHAPTER – Cross Training Equipment

I've been getting hundreds of emails every week asking what barbells, ropes and general equipment I recommend individuals use during their workouts, well by popular demand here is the Ultimate Cross Training WOD Equipment Guide!

It's imperative that you select high quality equipment that won't bend, break, fray or fall apart during intense workouts.

Eliminate the guess work and check out my Ultimate Cross Training WOD Equipment Guide available at:

www.shredded-society.com/Resources

These are the only pieces of equipment I use during my WODs, and these are the exact brands and items I use.

The equipment I own and use includes:

Olympic barbell

Your Olympic barbell is by far the most important piece of equipment you will own and use, it's the foundation of all major lifts.
When buying a barbell it's essential to check the weight rating – we don't want a cheap bar that is going to bend, it needs to stand the test of time. The bar is to have Olympic knurling, not powerlifting knurling.
Ensure the collars provided are sufficient.

Bumper Plates

High quality bumper plates are a must, if you train in your garage or anywhere at home for that matter damaging the flooring with regular plates is a common issue.

Pull Up Bar

Let's face it, many of us don't have room for a power station, and the majority of portable pull up bars out there are cheap and nasty or require a lot of drilling and doorway modifications.Luckily, I stumbled upon the Iron Gym Total Upper Body Workout Bar – no screws required!

Jump Rope

Skipping is fantastic cardio conditioning, a large amount of people skip daily, and most of those individuals tend to skimp on the quality of their jump rope – the Valeo Deluxe Speed Rope is adjustable, ideal for speed training and has the most comfortable handles on a jump rope I've encountered! If you want to smash out countless double-unders this is the rope for you!

Battling Rope

Battling ropes are optional, however they certainly do offer one of the most intense forms of cardio you'll experience. Battling ropes can be used to build immense shoulder and forearm strength.
I personally use a GoFit Combat Rope, comfortable handles, no fraying and can easily be anchored.

Gymnastic Rings

If you want to perform ring dips, push ups, muscle-ups and many other gymnastic style exercises a high quality set of rings are a must. The ProSource rings I use and recommend are made of premium quality Lexan and have a 1,000lb break strength.

Kettlebells

Kettlebells are a huge part of cross training. Want to swing, snatch or clean? you're going to need to pick up a couple of kettlebells!
I've gone through many kettlebells and the main issue I have

encountered is the seam on the underside of the handle, the majority of cheap kettlebells have a casting seam on the underside which will damage your hands.

Medicine/Slam Ball

Medicine balls are very versatile, want to perform wallballs, want to add weight to your push ups, planks or other core exercises? Want to play catch with a friend?

Ab Roller

Forget the ab swing pro and crunch king, whatever those crappy abdominal infomercial products are.
Invest in a high quality ab roller, the one abdominal training apparatus that only delivers results, no false promises.
I personally use the Ab Carver Pro, it features a kinetic engine, ultra wide wheel and a comfy foam knee pad!

Plyometric Box

If you're not a handyman and don't want to DIY your own plyometric box the Fuel Pureformance adjustable plyo box is a godsend! With 3 adjustable heights, a non slip surface and quick spring adjustment it's the Rolls Royce of plyometric boxes!

Minimalist Shoes

Running shoes are for running, not Olympic lifts or cross training in general.
You'll be surprised at how different performing lifts like the squat and deadlift in the correct cross training shoes.
New Balance have got these shoes down to a science with their 'Minimus' series.

Gloves

If you choose to wear gloves to stop your hands from getting ripped out during a workout it is quite hard to find the right pair that won't actually hinder your workout, the following gloves will keep your hands light, cool and protected throughout your workout – I cannot recommend these enough.

Wrist Wraps

Protect your wrists during heavy wraps, wear wrist straps.
These wrist wraps are high quality, reasonably priced and come with a no-hassle warranty.

Timer

As I'm sure you've noticed the majority of cross training workouts work on timed intervals, therefore an accurate timer is a must! After using and getting frustrated using a watch I decided to invest in a dedicated Everlast timer and have not looked back since.

Water Bottle

Staying hydrated during your workout is crucial for your health and well-being not to mention your performance during your workout.
Don't be one of those people that reuses an old plastic water bottle, they're known to cause a plethora of health issues when constantly reused.

I personally use and recommend a high quality Nalgene BPA free 1-quart bottle.

As mentioned above, for the links to each of the above products I recommend be sure to navigate to www.shredded-society.com/Resources

Conclusion

I hope you enjoy the plethora of bodyweight this book has to offer you, by following these workouts on a regular basis you'll develop not only a strong, flexible, functionally fit body that'll be ready to tackle any situation life throws at it but also an unbreakable mindset and confidence to match.

Whether you're looking to get a competitive advantage in your sport or just to increase your mobility, strength and health these workouts are the answer.

I hope you enjoyed reading this book as much as I enjoyed writing it.

Made in the USA
San Bernardino, CA
29 September 2015